THE HISTORY OF
HEMOSTASIS

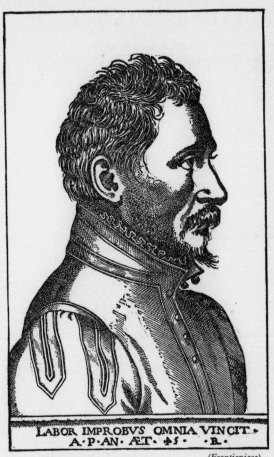

LABOR IMPROBVS OMNIA VINCIT·
A·P·AN·ÆT·45· ·B·

FIG. 1. AMBROISE PARÉ, AT THE AGE OF FORTY-FIVE.
(Anatomie Universelle, 1561.)

THE HISTORY OF
HEMOSTASIS

BY
SAMUEL CLARK HARVEY, M.D.
Professor of Surgery, Yale University;
Surgeon in Chief, New Haven Hospital

WITH 19 ILLUSTRATIONS

PAUL B · HOEBER · Inc
NEW YORK   MCMXXIX

Printed in the United States of America

TO
WILLIAM H. CARMALT
WHO IN HIS LIFE
HAS EXEMPLIFIED THE BEST
TRADITIONS OF SURGERY

PREFACE

THE fabric of history is made of the warp and woof of life and circumstance which seen as a whole forms a pattern of progress and retrogression so blended and intermingled that the casual student gains no clear concept of the texture. Biography is one fascinating method of analysis, the study of a period another, and a third the choosing of some theme and following it through the vicissitudes of time. In this *obiter opus* in medical history, the control of hemorrhage has been chosen as the thread to be followed amidst the varying fortunes of surgery.

In doing this, like Democritus Junior, I have gathered "wax and honey out of many flowers," the naming of which would give an appearance of erudition quite beyond the truth.

It is but justice, however, to express my grateful indebtedness to the writings of Allbutt, always so urbane and informative, particularly the essay on ".The Historical Relations of Medicine and Surgery," which the physician as well as the surgeon may still inwardly digest with profit to his soul. Likewise his "Greek Medicine in Rome" together with Charles Singer's discussion of medicine in Gilbert Murray's "The Legacy of Greece" bring home to us the extraordinary intellectual vitality of the Greek which should be our heritage. Neuburger, Gurlt and Sarton, as well as our own Garrison rest inevitably at one's elbow in such a search and a host of other witnesses not less worthy, the discovery of whom is no small part of the fun in historical browsing.

S. C. H.

New Haven, Connecticut
March, 1929

CONTENTS

LIST OF ILLUSTRATIONS

LIST OF ILLUSTRATIONS

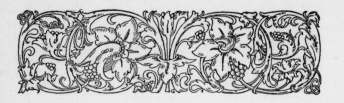

I

INTRODUCTION

THE history of surgery is largely written in the record of its technical advances. The greater of these have led to the control of pain, bleeding and infection and without these techniques the progress of surgery in the past half century would have been impossible. The development of antisepsis and asepsis is still a matter of the memory of the present generation, and anesthesia, in origin scarcely two decades older, has been repeatedly reviewed by those who had to do with its birth. Hemostasis, on the contrary, has been a matter of slow growth, keeping pace with the advancing knowledge of anatomy and physiology and reaching its present-day perfection in conjunction with anesthesia and asepsis. It has received but fragmentary and casual historical consideration.

The flow of blood following a wound is a phenomenon, the importance of which is apparent even to many animals. In attack, certain points at which to strike are selected instinctively and in defense likewise such areas are protected. However, any process of ratiocination directed toward the induction or control of hemorrhage is scarcely to be expected, though Pliny, the younger, credited the hippopotamus with such intelligence that it bled itself by thrusting a hollow reed into a vein. It may be more readily believed as stated by Neuburger "that monkeys seek to check the flow of blood by applications of the paw."

Although primitive man may have had no clearer notion of the phenomenon of bleeding than his progenitors, it excited his interest as did anything unusual about himself or about his environment. When the hunter slew his game or the warrior his foe, death came quickly when the purple tide freely flowed and as the dark blood clotted the spirit fled from its earthly abode. With the primitive man's crude reasoning by association, blood became the expression of the ghostly dangers with which he was hedged about and a starting point for magic, taboo and myth. So, according to Moses:

The priest shall sprinkle the blood upon the altar of the Lord at the door of the tabernacle of the congregation, and, whatsoever man hunteth and catcheth any beast or fowl that may be eaten; he shall even pour out the blood thereof, and cover it with dust. For it is the life of all flesh.

The apotheosis of superstition was reached in the ritual of Attis at

Rome which Frazer, in "The Golden Bough," describes as follows:

In the baptism the devotee, crowned with gold and wreathed with fillets, descended into a pit, the mouth of which was covered with a wooden grating. A bull, adorned with garlands of flowers, its forehead glittering with gold leaf, was then driven on to the grating and there stabbed to death with a consecrated spear. Its hot reeking blood poured in torrents through the apertures, and was received with devout eagerness by the worshipper on every part of his person and garments, till he emerged from the pit, drenched, dripping, and scarlet from head to foot, to receive the homage, nay the adoration, of his fellows as one who had been born again to eternal life and had washed away his sins in the blood of the bull.

This superstitious respect for blood so thoroughly enmeshed science and surgery with the black thread of magic and the red skein of religion, that a thousand years was scarcely sufficient to disentangle them.

Nevertheless, the exigencies of warfare, of the hunt and of daily toil, made necessary some attempt at hemostasis. The epics of early Greece and Rome portrayed again and again the fleeting of the vital spirits with the pouring out of the blood and attempts were made to prevent this. When Menelaus was shot through the belt, the treatment was as follows: "The godlike hero Machaeon drew then forth the arrow from golden haired Menelaus and sucked out the blood from the wound and cunningly spread thereon soothing drugs, such as Cheiron of his good will had imparted to his son."

In the Aeneid:

Venus for her darling filled with grief
A stalk of dittany of Ida's crown
Seeks out, and gathers, for his wound's relief,
The flower of purple and the leaves of down.
(To wounded wild-goats 'twas a plant well-
    known).
This brings the Goddess, veiled in mist, and
    brews
In a bright bowl a mixture of her own,

And, steeped in water from the stream, she
strews
Soft balm of fragrant scent, and sweet
ambrosial dews.
Therewith the leech, unwitting, rinsed the
wound,
And the pain fled, and all the blood was
stayed.

In a general if poetical manner, this
portrays the degree of knowledge of
the Greek of the Homeric period and
corresponds to that employed by
uncivilized man in various parts of the
world today. According to Neuburger:
"Arrest of hemorrhage presents great
difficulties to aborigines, for the most
part they do not know how to attack
it. It is sometimes brought about by
means of vegetable and mineral styptics, less often it is attempted by
means of circular pressure (tightly
bound bandages)."

II

THE BEGINNINGS OF HEMOSTASIS

When the Greeks, as recounted in Herodotus, encountered Egyptian medicine, it was in its decline, probably having reached its zenith some 1300 years previously. The Ebers' Papyrus described operative procedures in which the danger of hemorrhage was recognized. "When thou feelest a fatty growth in the neck and feelest it like an abscess of the flesh and soft to the fingers, then sayest thou, 'He has a fatty growth on his neck, I will treat the disease with the knife, *paying heed to the vessels.*'"

They also employed as medicaments lead sulphate, antimony, verdegris and copper sulphate, the last of which we shall recognize later as the "hemostatic button." In India, venesection was practiced and bleeding was controlled by elevation, cold, compression, and hot oil. Among the Chinese, hemorrhage was arrested by styptics and bandaging. All the civilizations in the first millennium before Christ—the Chinese, the Indian, the Assyrio-Babylonian and the Egyptian —were at much the same level as regards surgery and in particular the control of hemorrhage. The progress of further knowledge was blocked by oriental formalism and mysticism, and as Allbutt says, it remained for the "lucid and positive intelligence of the Greeks to transfer this into unimportant mythology and to apply the rational mind to the study of Medicine."

Alcmaion of Crotona, a contemporary of Pythagoras, distinguished in the cadaver between empty veins and veins containing blood; and Diogenes of Appollonia (*ca.* 430 B.C.) was among the earliest to describe blood vessels but supposed that they carried air to the different parts of the

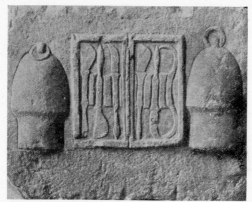

Fig. 2. Cases Containing Scalpels and Tenaculum. Bleeding Cups on Either Side. Pre-Hippocratic Monumental Carving.

(From Sudhoff-Meyer-Steineg.)

system. He did not recognize the heart as the starting point of the vessels. These, the first gropings of the pre-Hippocratic group, come down to us through Aristotle, for their writings, apparently voluminous, have otherwise disappeared.

In the corpus Hippocraticum, which was written in the main between 400 and 300 B.C. the "blood is the chief material from which organs are built up; it is produced in the liver and obtains the necessary temperature in the left ventricle. From there propelled by the pulsating heart, it circulates by means of the veins throughout the entire body." The content of the left ventricle and of the arteries was supposed to be either pneuma alone or principally pneuma with only the smallest particles of blood. The proof of this was the emptiness of the left ventricle at death, the hissing sound when an artery was sectioned, and the steaming of the blood as it poured out upon the ground. This unfortunate doctrine of the pneuma, hypothesized by Empedocles and Pythagoras among others in an effort to find some method of circulation for the spirit of life itself, was passed onward through Aristotle and Galen, until it became the "quintessence" of Harvey, the "phlogiston" of Black and the "oxygen" of Lavoisier; finally leaving the name "artery" as a lone relic of a discarded philosophy. It is not surprising to find that the Hippocratic operations were largely those which could be performed without hemostasis. Ligation of vessels was unknown and amputations done only through the gangrenous extremity below the zone of demarcation. Such means as were used for controlling accidental hemorrhage were various styptics, elevation and compression, tamponage and bandage and infrequently the cautery.

The reasoning mind of the Greek followed the Alexandrian armies into Asia Minor, Egypt, and as far abroad as the Punjab; and Ptolemy founded

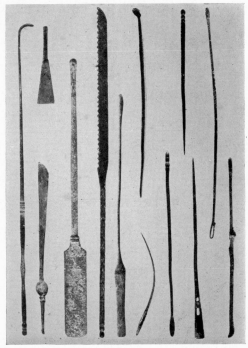

FIG. 3. SURGICAL INSTRUMENTS OF HIPPOCRATIC
TIMES. TENACULUM ON LEFT.
(FROM SUDHOFF-MEYER-STEINEG.)

the Alexandrian library, drawing there
the best of Greek culture including
that in medicine and surgery. The
custom of embalming, a religious rite,
had made the Egyptians familiar with
dissection of the human body. It
was but a short step from this to
purposeful dissection and the first
respectable knowledge of anatomy
was acquired at this time. Hero-
philus "with great care described
the course relationship of the vascular
system and distinguished the blood
conducting veins from the arteries,
filled with blood and pneuma, which
arose from the heart and possess
coats six times as strong." Erasistratus
described the heart with its valves
and chordae tendineae and thought
that the arteries (containing pneuma)
had their origin in the heart: "From
the liver where blood first comes into
existence, it is conducted into the
venae cavae and is distributed by the
way of the venous system." He also
hypothecated the capillary circulation
as "synanastomoses" which under

normal circumstances were closed, though when an artery was cut, blood might penetrate through these into the arterial circulation, following the escape of the pneuma, the response being due to the law of *natura abhorret vacuum*. Hemorrhage then did not come directly from arteries, but indirectly through the "synanasto-moses" and arrest of bleeding consequently might cause a plethora in the arterial system, a supposedly undesirable thing. The pneuma of the philosophers still befogged the observations of the anatomists and: "bombastic plausibility and craziness flaunting as erudition, in the end won the day against the homely truth of plain hands and honest eyes." The momentary brilliancy of Alexandria was soon obscured by pedantic erudition and by oriental mysticism drifting in from the East.

III

THE GRECO-ROMANS

"After the destruction of Corinth (146 B.C.)," as Garrison says, "Greek medicine . . . migrated to Rome," where the atmosphere of pragmatic practicality seems to have served surgery well. From this time, until Galen (some three hundred years) was a golden age in surgery, but unfortunately the literature of it is in large part extinct and dependence must be had upon the compilations of Celsus, Oribasius, and Paul of Aegina, with argumentative references in Galen. Celsus advanced beyond the Hippocratic doctrine to the point of amputation at the line of demarcation, where in most instances the vessels would be already occluded. Even at that, *in ipso opere, vel profusione sanguinis, vel animae dejectione moriuntur.* While not using the ligature in the amputation stump, he did propose the pulling up of the vessel in a wound, ligating it on either side of the injured point and completing the division, although he recommended the trial of compression and styptics first. Ligature was then a matter of last resort and not of election and the use of it probably infrequent and confined to accidental wounds. Heliodorus used a bandage about the limb above the site of amputation in order, so far as possible, to bring about the closure of the vessels. He described amputation through the lower leg but it is doubtful if he carried out any amputation of election above the knee or elbow.

Archigenes (*ca.* 100 A.D.) was more daring and advanced the scope of practice materially. He proposed amputating in "gangrene, necrosis, cancer, and certain callus tumors." As a preliminary he suggested that the vessels leading to the site of amputation be tied, bound or sewn but it is

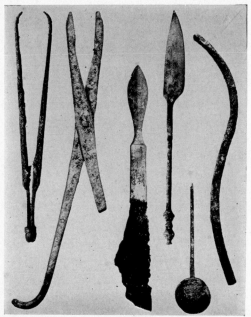

Fig. 4. Surgical Instruments of Early Roman Times. On Left a Depilator and Directly Adjacent Forceps for Drawing Teeth.

(From Sudhoff-Meyer-Steineg.)

doubtful if this meant ligation of arteries in continuity. The knowledge of the anatomical landmarks of the great vessels was too indefinite, the veins were supposed to contain the blood and the arteries only pneuma and a double operative procedure would have been improbable. The soft parts were retracted, the skin first, then the "tendon" so as to give a properly covered stump. The cautery and the usual styptics were applied to control bleeding.[1] Soranus,

[1] There seems to be a considerable confusion concerning the practice of the time in this respect. Garrison says: "Heliodorus, who antedated Celsus, gave the first account of ligation and torsion of blood vessels." It is not usually stated that Heliodorus did antedate Celsus, for he is mentioned by Juvenal and has been supposed to have been contemporaneous with this author (*ca.* 100 A.D.), while Celsus wrote nearly one hundred years earlier. He recommended the ligation and torsion of vessels (after excising the dartos) in operating for hernia and not in the operation of amputation. In this respect he was in entire accord with Celsus who probably did not practice but was an unusually able com-

who wrote greatly on obstetrics, gyne-
cology and pediatrics, recommended
the division of the cord by the knife
and the use of the ligature if the
placenta was still attached. Rufus of
Ephesus, a few years preceding Galen
wrote in the same sense as Archigenes,
recommending the arrest of hemorrhage by digital pressure, pressure
with bandages, cold, astringents, tor-

---

piler and who described the same methods of
handling hemorrhage in accidental wounds.
In all probability the introduction of the
ligation of damaged vessels was a matter of
the Alexandrian school for the corpus Hippocraticum has nothing to say of it.

Allbutt, as well as other recent writers,
has stated that Archigenes used the ligature in
amputation. This seems to have been based
upon the section in Oribasius which was
copied from the writings, long since vanished,
of this remarkable surgeon. The original
Greek is difficult of translation but probably
referred to types of bandages applied above
the amputation site to compress the veins
rather than to ligation in continuity or in
the stump as has been assumed by some.
Certainly the tourniquet was not used as has
been suggested.

sion and ligature, and severance of incised vessels. With the ligation of vessels in a wound the application of a similar procedure to aneurysm by Antyllus was but a natural step. He described the occurrence of both the spontaneous and the traumatic aneurysm and recommended the ligation on either side of the tumor and the evacuation of its contents by incision. That this could have been successfully applied to the large aneurysm with its many and large collateral vessels running directly into the sac is improbable and indeed this author, as well as Galen, advises against the attempt in tumors of the groin, axilla and at the base of the neck.

The period in which these men worked, a matter of three hundred years, was the golden age of Rome so well described by Gibbon, in the opening chapters of the "Decline and Fall." It was a period of opulence and power for the few, of poverty and degradation for the many, but withal

a time of freedom of thought insofar
as it did not conflict with the political
hegemony. For the medical sciences
it was the second day of light and
growth flaring out at the last in Galen.

As a philosopher, Galen dispersed
the pneuma of Erasistratus but suc-
ceeded in fixing vitalism on medicine
until the present day; as an anatomist
he systematized and amplified the
anatomy of Alexandria but derived
his knowledge from animals, not men;
and as a compiler he brought the
medical knowledge of his time into an
encyclopedia, including the surgery
of Antyllus, Soranus, Rufus and
Archigenes. As a physiologist, he
showed by means of vivisection that
the arteries contained blood and not
air and missed the correct description
of the circulation and the true action
of the heart by a narrow margin.
Though his description and practice
in surgery are detailed and precise,
it is probable that he actually did but
little surgery. As regards the control
of hemorrhage he was dependent upon

the work of his immediate predeces-
sors. When blood was discharged
from a wounded artery, a finger was
applied to the orifice of the vessel
firmly, yet not so as to occasion pain,
and then a thrombus would form
that would stop the flow of blood.
When the vessel was deeply seated he
advised one to examine accurately
into the situation and size and to
ascertain whether it was an artery or
vein; after which it was to be seized
with a hook and twisted moderately.
If the flow of blood was not stopped
thereby, and if the vessel was a vein,
an endeavor was made to restrain it
without a ligature by means of styptics or things of an obstruent nature
such as roasted rosin, the fine down
of wheat and flour, gypsum and the
like. But if the vessel was an artery,
one of two things must be done:
either a ligature must be applied to it,
or it must be cut across. As a ligature,
he recommended Celtic linen, probably obtained from Scotland, and
named the shop in the Via Sacra in

which it might be bought. Although completely familiar with ligation in the accidental wound, he did not mention its use in amputations. In fact his descriptions of this procedure were without detail.

IV

THE CAUTERY

After Galen, as Allbutt says, "begins the night"—a long one—"of the second day." He died at the close of the second century shortly after the exitus of his patron, the flower of the Emperors, Marcus Aurelius. Within a little over one hundred years, a century of internal dissension, superstition and fanaticism, the great persecution of Diocletian had failed and Constantine officially Christianized the Roman Empire. With the apostasy of Julian and perhaps as a result of his furore for Paganism, Oribasius wrote his compendium of the medicine of antiquity from which most of our information back as far as the corpus Hippocraticum is derived. This was but a flash and the overturning of the Western Empire by the barbarians and the domination of the Eastern Empire by Byzantine courtiers and religious fanatics put an end to all advance in medicine. Gregory the Great became the first pope in 590 A.D. and the church assumed complete control of all thought. Aetius of Amida and Alexander of Tralles in the sixth century and Paul of Aegina in the seventh century were compilers, to whose originality we owe nothing but who with Galen were carried over into the Arabian school and there served to link the Middle Ages with antiquity. In the surgery of the blood vessels they did little but quote the ancients and in the compilations of Paul of Aegina, it is apparent that the standards of practice had made no advance since the first century.

Meanwhile the strife within the church was bearing its fruit. Nestor, the patriarch of Constantinople, had been deposed in 428 A.D., and driven first to Edessa and later into Persia. The Nestorians carried with them the yeast of Greek culture which leavened the great Arabian movement and found its way across Egypt, Northern Africa, the Straits of Gibraltar, through Cordova and at last, in the tenth century, into Italy. Joannitius, "the Erasmus of the Arabic renaissance" in the ninth century translated Hippocrates, Galen, Oribasius and Paul into Arabic and therewith formed the groundwork for Rhazes, Avicenna and Albucasis, the great compilers and practitioners of Arabian medicine.

These men, in surgery, did little but apply the sayings of the ancients and in particular this is true of hemostasis. The measure of their prowess is found in Albucasis (eleventh century) whose text was authoritative in western surgery until the time of Guy de Chauliac, or the middle of the fourteenth century. Surgery had become an inferior and separate branch of medicine, as implied by Avicenna and the cautery had in large part replaced the knife. True, the ligation of vessels was

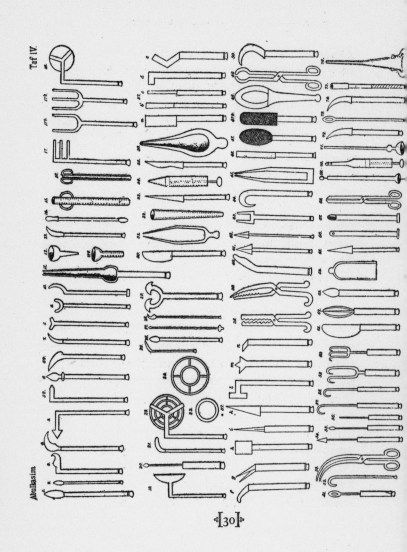

advised by Paul—Paré used Avicenna
as an authority for his method—but
cauterization was the common procedure, refined in its cruelty and
explicit in its application. It is somewhat difficult to understand this
depreciation.

The practice of cauterization had
derived authoritative support from
Hippocrates and Galen. According to
the former: "that what the medicament quelleth not, the iron doth; and
that which the iron amendeth not, the
fire extermineth." In every treatise
the cautery was recommended when
everything else failed and such was
usually the situation at once in amputation. It was not within the province
of the oriental mind to question such
dicta. That same mind was warped
by the taboo of the East as regards
defilement by contact with the body

FIG. 5. SURGICAL INSTRUMENTS AS ILLUSTRATED IN
ALBUCASIS. MANY CAUTERIES OF VARYING FORMS. 31
AND 45 ARE DEPILATION OR TISSUE FORCEPS. 38, 39
AND 53 ARE DENTAL FORCEPS ADAPTED FOR REMOVAL
OF FOREIGN BODIES. 53 IS "BEC DE CORBIN" OF PARÉ.
(FROM GURLT.)

or with the blood. Surgery, degraded by this superstition—in fact, as a profession, largely wiped out—was confined to the treatment of wounds. Anatomical knowledge and manual dexterity were in abeyance and when most needed were lacking. Anyone could apply the cautery, practically no one the ligature.

Albucasis had this to say concerning the control of bleeding in a wound:

Arterial hemorrhage is frequently seen following the rupture of an artery in wounds from external causes, in the opening of a swelling, in the cauterization of an organ and in other similar circumstances. If you find yourself in this situation, apply promptly the hand over the opening in the vessel, press with the index finger until the blood is stopped under your finger and flows forth no more. Put on the fire an assortment of olivary cauteries and blow upon them until they are well heated. Take one of them, large or small, according to the size and shape of the part where the artery is ruptured. Apply the cautery on the artery itself, after having quickly raised the finger and hold it there until the bleeding is stopped.

As regards amputation, he performed it only as high as the elbow or knee. He says: "if during the operation an hemorrhage occurs, cauterize promptly or apply an hemostatic powder." Otherwise the procedure differs in no way from that of the ancients.

V

HEMOSTASIS IN THE WESTERN
WORLD

Saracen culture was then in considerable part responsible for the backwardness of surgery in the west and its influence lasted for some five centuries. The educated class in Italy and in France was in large part ecclesiastic, that is to say scholastic, and spent their time arguing, like Abelard, for Platonic nominalism or like St. Thomas Aquinas for Aristotelian realism. Logic was chopped, sophistry was knowledge, and observation and trial by experimentation unknown. The use of the hands except for the gestures of oratory was undignified and operative skill was the property of the itinerant quack who became so great an evil that all surgery, except that done by clerics, was wisely forbidden. However, the shedding of blood, a mystery of Attis as described previously, had curiously interwoven itself with the mysticism of the early church so that it soon became taboo in the only class which was qualified by knowledge to carry it out. The council of Tours in 1163 promulgated the doctrine *ecclesia abhorret a sanguine* and surgery was at an end in the educated class and interdicted among the uneducated. It is not surprising then that it remained largely a matter of the treatment of wounds and that the control of hemorrhage followed faithfully the methods laid down in the Arabian texts.

There came after a time, however, certain independent minds, who learned from observation, such as Hugh of Lucca and his pupil Theodoric who believed in healing *per primam* and used the suture and ligature in hemorrhage. Saliceto in the early thirteenth century restored the use of the knife and diagnosed arterial bleeding by the spurting of the blood. Lanfranc, the father of

French surgery in the latter part of the same century, differentiated arterial from venous bleeding and treated hemorrhage by styptics, compresses, torsion and even the ligature. He was in the main, however, a cauterist; in fact, the more of a scholar the greater the use of the cautery, was in general the rule. Henri de Mondeville, of the same period, but more educated by his hands felt that "God did not exhaust all the creative power in making Galen" and used styptics, digital compression, acupressure, torsion and ligation of isolated vessels by means of a sliding noose ligature. The importance to the surgeon of anatomy had again begun to be recognized, for Guy de Chauliac said that the surgeon ignorant of anatomy, "carves the human body as a sculptor carves wood." So dissection was started at Montpellier and Mundinus wrote the first anatomy in 1316.

The fifteenth century is notable for many things including the popu-

larization of the use of gunpowder
and the development of the art of
printing. Marcello seems to have
been first to write of the treatment
of gunshot wounds, while a confrère,
Leonardo Bertopaglia, a professor at
Padua, investigated the indications
for and the methods of application
of the ligature. He drew the vessel
forward with a steel hook, isolated
it and tied it with a flaxen thread,
twisting the thread first, to make fast
the knots. He sutured wounds of the
intestine with a glover's stitch and
used softened catgut in preference
to thread for the purpose, a method
recommended previously by Rhazes.
He did not, however, apply it in
amputations. It must be remembered
that such knowledge as these men
had was acquired by very rare, incom-
plete and hasty dissections and by
the perusal of frequently copied manu-
scripts. With the advent of printing,
knowledge became at once much more
universal and accessible. The classics
were printed, particularly the trans-

lations from the Arabic, and the Mundinus anatomy appeared in 1473. Guy's surgery went into many editions and became widely distributed. John of Vigo (1514) wrote the surgery of this time, authoritative particularly in regard to gunshot wounds. Amputation for injury was described, still with the use of the cautery, while the ligature was applied only in the manner of Celsus. Gunshot wounds were poisoned "a priori" and Ambroise Paré attempted to carry John of Vigo's methods into practice.

VI

PARÉ AND THE LIGATURE

Paré was untrained in the classics.
Indeed, it is doubtful if he could read
anything but the vernacular. He derived his knowledge by dissection
and by service as a dresser in the
wards of the Hôtel Dieu and as a
surgeon on the battlefield. He broke
away from servility to tradition and
allowed his keen and untrammeled
intelligence to carry him into new
practices. Of chief interest here is
the development of his methods in
the control of hemorrhage.

In 1537 when Paré received his
baptism in war surgery there seemed
many cogent reasons for the cauterization of wounds, either by hot oil
or by the use of the actual cautery.
All the ancients agreed upon this
procedure. It was assumed that all

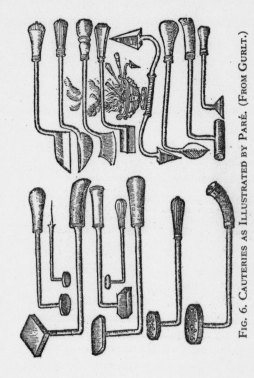

Fig. 6. Cauteries as Illustrated by Paré. (From Gurlt.)

gunshot wounds were poisoned and that the natural process was toward gangrene. As Paré says: "They partook of a venomous nature." However, he in his first war experience was soon pressed for lack of the particular oil in use and was forced to dress the wound with a "digestive" of the yolk of eggs, the oil of olives and turpentine. He says:

That night I could not sleep at ease, fearing by lack of cauterization, that I should find the wounded, on whom I had failed to put the said oil, dead or empoisoned, which made me rise very early to visit them. When beyond my hope, I found them upon whom I had put the digestive medicament feeling little pain and their wounds without inflammation or swelling having rested fairly well throughout the night. Then I resolved with myself never more to burn thus cruelly poor men wounded with gunshot.

For fifteen years afterward he must have been turning over in his mind the possibility of likewise avoiding the use of the cautery in amputations.

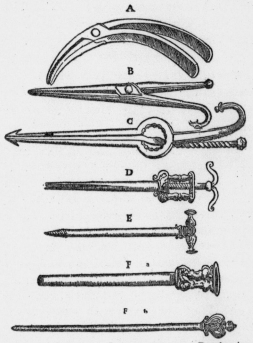

FIG. 7. SURGICAL INSTRUMENTS OF PARÉ. A IS
"BEC DE CORBIN" WITH WHICH HE GRASPED BLEED-
ING VESSEL IN ORDER TO LIGATE IT. (FROM GURLT.)

Meanwhile he persistently continued his dissections and in 1549 published a small anatomy. He was well aware of the statements of the authorities as regards the ligation of vessels in wounds but scarcely dared extend the method to amputations. At last in 1552, he amputated the leg of an officer who had been wounded at the siege of Danvilliers, using the ligature instead of hot irons to check the hemorrhage. "I dressed him and God healed him. He returned home gaily with a wooden leg, saying that he had got off cheaply without being miserably burned to stop the bleeding."

After this performance the next edition of his "Dix Livres de la Chirurgie" which appeared in 1564 advised the abandonment of the cautery altogether. Twenty years later Etienne Gourmelen, dean of the faculty of medicine of Paris, made himself famous by virulently attacking this procedure and to him we are indebted for Paré's delightful rejoinder, the "Apology and Journeys." In this

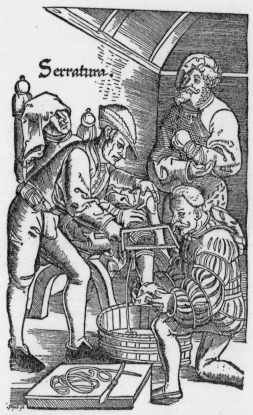

FIG. 8. FIRST ILLUSTRATION OF AMPUTATION, FROM
VON GERSDORFF (1517). BANDAGES CONSTRICT, AT
MOST, SUPERFICIAL VEINS. TWO ARTERIES ARE
SPURTING UNCONTROLLED. MAN IN BACKGROUND IS
WEARING GERSDORFF'S PIG'S BLADDER DRESSING
OVER HIS FOREARM STUMP.

we learn considerably more concerning his practice. He amputated above the portion mortified and corrupted, returning to the practice of Archigenes.

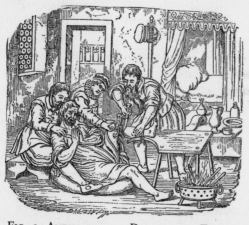

Fig. 9. Amputation as Depicted by Fabricius Hildanus (1593). Assistant Is Using Compression Bandage above Incision for Retraction of Stump. Irons which Fabricius Recommended for Amputation are at Hand in Charcoal Salamander.

He thought it not necessary "to use fire—to consume and check the putrefaction which is common to gangrenous mortifications." He drew the bleeding vessel forth by grasping it with a "bec de corbin" (a bullet

[45]

grasping instrument), which therefore became the true ancestor of the artery forceps. Previously vessels had been handled with a hook or tenaculum, and then only in wounds and not in amputation stumps. Now for the first time a vessel was caught with a pinching instrument which would control the bleeding while it was being handled. He gave five case histories, in which the ligature was used, four of amputations below the knee and one probably below the elbow. He ligated *en masse* but the material of the ligature was not mentioned or whether he cut the thread short or left it hanging from the wound.

The adoption of Paré's suggestion was far from immediate, although his opinion was frequently quoted and tentatively recommended. Even his pupil Guillemeau (1602) adopted a middle attitude between "les deux grands personnages de nostre temps, l'un medecin, l'autre chieurgen" and reserved the ligature for amputation through healthy tissue. Where the incision was carried across vessels that might be diseased he feared that the ligature would cut through and employed the cautery. In general, he agreed with Paré that amputation should be carried through healthy tissue above the diseased portion of the limb. Fallopius (1606), the teacher of Harvey at Padua, thanked God that he had the audacity to use the ligature in the control of hemorrhage but his daring did not carry him as far as amputations. In his description of this operation he recommended the use of the cautery. Fabricius ab Aquapendente, in the "Pentateuch" (1617) did not mention the use of the ligature whereas Dalechamp (1573) briefly called attention to Paré's procedure with no comment as to its effectiveness. Rauchin (1580) in a similar treatise recommended Paré's procedure without giving credit for it. Schenck (1643) gave impartially Paré's description and Gourmelen's criticism. His was a compilation of previous writers, the product of a scholar and not that of a practitioner in surgery.

Fabricius Hildanus (1615) in the standard German text of his time wrote a classical description of amputation with no reference to Paré's method. Sennert in 1620 mentioned Paré's method only to condemn it and summed up the objections in a similar manner to Gourmelen—the procedure was difficult, time consuming and dangerous and that when accomplished it led to fever, with the additional danger of puncturing the adjacent nerve which would result in convulsions and great danger to life.

The primary determining factor at this period as to the use of the ligature was the type of amputation employed. As we have seen, many of the great writers recommended amputation according to the Hippocratic method; that is, through the diseased tissues. Others suggested the method of Celsus, which was carrying the amputation through or adjacent to the line of demarcation. Relatively few, of whom Archigenes and Paré were notable examples, advised amputation above the diseased portion of the limb and through healthy tissue. It is apparent that the latter group would find the control of hemorrhage with the cautery difficult and would naturally tend to use the ligature, while the former group would have less difficulty because the vessels would be frequently already thrombosed.

In the English literature, Thomas Gale (1563) does not refer to ligature of the vessels but Clowes (1596) who wrote in French, but of whom an English translation appeared in 1637, quotes Guillemeau, Paré's pupil, in favor of ligation. He, however, adds: "I have practiced this order by attaching the veins and arteries. I will leave it as aforesaid and proceed with mine own approved practice."

Lowe (1597) says: "cut rather a little of the whole, rather than leave any portion of the infected—where there is no putrefaction, malignancy nor humor venemous we use the ligator." Lowe practiced surgery for twenty-two years in France and Flanders, and for two years was surgeon major to the Spanish regiments in Paris (1589–90). From 1596–98 he was in London and in the latter year founded the School of Medicine in Glasgow. His "A Discourse of the Whole Art of Chyrurgery" London, 1596, represented the first adequate description in English of the best of the French practice. In regard to amputation he says:

I advise to make the incision four inches from the joynt in all amputations, except only when the mortification on riving of the bone end in the joynt, then it must be cut in the joynt, chiefly the joynt of the knee; always it is hard to ciccatrize and heal, by reason the end of the bone is spongious and humid, so the loather to conglutinate; but wheresoever you make your amputation, remember to mark it well with ink or others, and to cut rather a little of the whol, then to leave any portion of the infected. If any of the

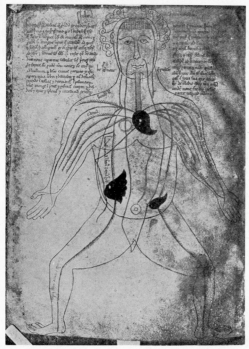

Fig. 10. Inadequate Depiction of Anatomy of
Peripheral Vessels, 13th Century. (De Lint.)

infected remain, it corrupteth the rest,
and so requireth new amputation, as I
have often seen . . . the chyurgion shall
pluck up the skinn and muscles as much
as he can, thereafter he shall take a strong
ribbon, and binde the member fast about
the place of the member, two inches abowe
where the amputation shall be . . . we
cut the flesh with a razor or incising knife,
which must be somewhat crooked though
the form of a hook or half moon . . . The
flesh then being so cut to the bone, the
said bone must be diligently rubbed and
scraped with the back of the sayd knife,
which back must be made purposely for
that effect, to the end of the periost which
covereth the bone, may be lesse painful in
cutting of the bone. Otherwise it teareth
and riveth with the same, so causeth
great dolour; Also letteth the cutting,
although the bone hath no feeling of
itself. This being done, you must saw the
bone with a sharpe sawe; then loose the
ligatour, draw down the skin, and cover
the bone in all the parts; and if there be
great putrefaction, let it bleed a little, for
that dischargeth the part and so is lesse
subject to inflammation: then one of the
assisters shall put the extreamities of his

fingers on the great veins and arteries, to stay them from bleeding, till the chyurgion either knit or cauterize them one after another, as he shall think expedient. But where there is putrefaction, we stay the flux of blood by cauters actuals, and where there is no putrefaction, malignitis, nor humor venemous, we use the ligator. The cauter or actuall fire maketh scale, stayeth bleeding, consumeth and draweth into it the virulency and malignitis of the humor which is in that part, and in that point it is more sure and better than knitting. In knitting we lose much blood, and by drawing the veins with back decurbing, or other instrument, they doe breake. Also being knit, doe often unloose, so that I find the fire more expedient, being done and applyed meanly. Then to doe it, we must have three or foure little instruments of iron, crooked at the end, with a point in form of a button; of which, some be round, some silate, and some broad, to rub on the end of the bone . . . It hath the virtue to dry and coroborate the same, being made red hot: then we take eyther of them and apply on the veines one after another, continuing them a certain space till the scale be made,

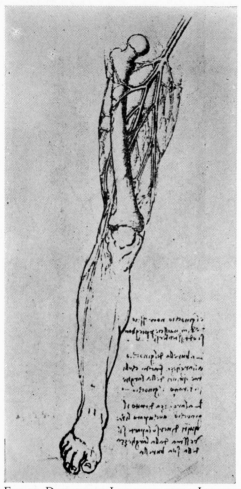

FIG. 11. DRAWING OF LEONARDO AFTER INJECTION OF VESSELS. DEPICTION IS STILL INADEQUATE AND CONFUSED (15TH CENTURY).

taking heed alwaies not to burn overmuch of the vein . . . In amputation without putrefaction, I find the ligator reasonable sure, providing it be quickly done. To doe it first thou shalt cause the assister as I have said, to hold his fingers on the veines, letting one loose, on the which thou shalt take hold with the back decurbin, taking a little of the flesh or muscles with it; then put through a needle with a strong thread, knit with a double knot, tying a little of the flesh with the veine, which will make it hold the better: but if it slip, as oft it happeneth, you shall first put through the needle in the utter skin, an inch above the wound, neere to the side of the vein, cause it to come forth by the other side of the vein, yet higher than the orifice of the veine: then pul out your needle an inch from the part where it went in, then put a piece of cloth in two doubles betwixt the two threads, then tye it hard, to the end the knot enter not in the skinne. This way and forme must be used in the rest of the veines, as also in divers other parts of the body."

Woodall in 1639 advocated the amputation "in the rotten part" saying that he had not lost a single patient of 100 so treated nor had the "mortification spread itself any further at all." It was of course not necessary to use the ligature.

The civil and religious discords of the seventeenth century in Germany, in France and in England seem to have held the advancement of surgery in abeyance. From Fabricius Hildanus to Petit no great name occurs among the surgeons and the work of the former remained the standard of practice for this time, being quoted by all authors even into the early part of the nineteenth century and serving in the German as a common text for the "Wund Arzt" until the time of Heister (1724). Meanwhile the basic sciences were thriving and particularly anatomy with its physiological correlations. The "De Motu Cordis" (1628) established the circulation of the blood and the exact distribution and relation of the arteries were shortly worked out. The fine copper plates of a little later (Bidloo, 1685) added to their exact delineation and refined methods of injecting vessels (Ruysch, 1655) enabled the anatomist to distinguish them from other structures aiding greatly in their accurate dissection. It was only a short step forward to the first modern text on anatomy, that of von Soemmerring (1791–96).

VII

THE TOURNIQUET

The "ligatures" of Archigenes and
Heliodorus were still used to control
the superficial vessels (veins) and to
benumb the skin. They consisted of
narrow bands of cloth placed directly
above and below the line of incision,
whipped two or three times about the
limb and tied in a single knot. The
first picture of an amputation, that of
von Gersdorff, shows how ineffectual
this was, for the two tibial arteries
appear spurting forcibly from the
stump through such a ligature or
bandage. It was necessary to act
hastily before the patient became
exsanguinated, particularly in amputation of the larger extremities. To
grasp a large vessel with the clumsy
"bec de corbin" of Paré, to draw it
out and transfix it with needle and

thread and then tie, required a precision of movement and a manual dexterity which was probably not

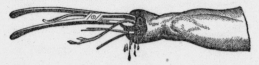

Fig. 12. The "Bec de Corbin" Applied as Illustrated by Guillemeau (1585). It Has Been Provided with Spring.

common. In clumsy hands the patient might die before the several vessels were successfully ligated. Consequently when Paré's method was advocated, it was directed that an assistant should control the other vessels by direct pressure in the wound, thus necessitating the presence of a second person to perform a necessarily clumsy and inefficient task.

Some time in this period, it is difficult to say when or by whom, it was discovered that compression applied over the great arterial trunks, proximally at some distance from the site of amputation, would control

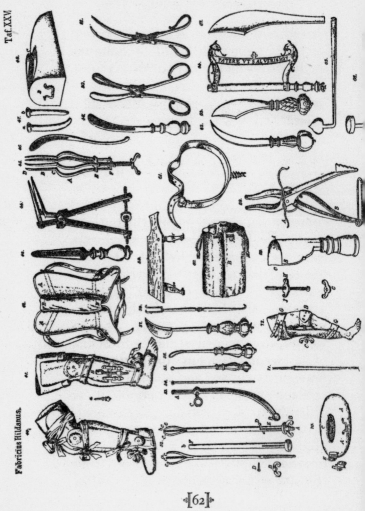

bleeding. The accurate localization of these vessels had now become known and was a matter of common knowledge to the well informed surgeon. Both Paré and Wiseman had mentioned the possibility of control by manupressure but added that this was ineffective because of the strength required. This application was not directed at precise digital control but general compression which could not be long maintained. There was then no effective temporary method of hemostasis and whatever procedure was applied had to be carried out in the presence of active bleeding. Morel in the siege of Besançon (1674) was, as far as can be determined, the first to introduce a stick into the upper bandage, and twist it until the arterial flow stopped, thus giving time for the securing of permanent hemostasis. This was a most important discovery; indeed, it

FIG. 13. SURGICAL INSTRUMENTS OF FABRICIUS HILDANUS. 68 REPRESENTS "BEC DE CORBIN" ALSO PROVIDED WITH CATCH AND ITS USE INDICATED BY LIGATURE CAST LOOSELY ABOUT IT.

is doubtful if the ligature in amputation could have won out as the method of choice, had it not been for this maneuver. The introduction of the tourniquet was rapid. Dionis (1707), who credited the invention to Morel, recommended it and Heister (1724) described its application and illustrated the procedure in his great surgery both in the upper and lower extremities. In these plates, small rolls of cloth were indicated beneath the tourniquet over the femoral and brachial arteries, an evidence of the application of the current anatomical and physiological knowledge. Further improvements of the tourniquet, such as Petit's screw tourniquet, the tourniquet of rubber tubing, the Esmarch bandage and the calliper tourniquet were unimportant compared with the establishment of the principle by Morel.

VIII

HEMOSTASIS IN THE 18TH CENTURY

The reign of the *Roi Soleil* in
France meant as much for surgery
as for the other arts which he patron-
ized. The cure by Felix of the royal
fistula-in-ano served to place the
French surgeon at a point of advantage as regards education so that
in the succeeding generation there
appeared the great French school of
the early eighteenth century, marked
by such names as Petit, Desault and
Chopart. Of this school all modern
surgery is the lineal descendant.

By surveying the work of these
men together with that of Cheselden
and Pott in England and Heister in
Germany, one may arrive at the
standard practice of the eighteenth
century. It is at once apparent that
the tourniquet had won the field. No

longer was there discussion of the problem of the staying of blood during the operation itself, nor was there any question as to the desirability of amputating above the disease. The Paré method had not clearly won out, however, for the chemical styptics ranked first, though the actual cautery is a poor third. The application of the tourniquet was described with precision but the ligature was reserved for the large vessels in amputations above the knee or elbow which were now for the first time generally attempted. The "vitriol or hemostatic button" was employed for medium sized vessels, alum for the still smaller and direct compression followed by bandaging for the smallest of all. The chemical styptic had displaced the actual cautery as well as the animal or vegetable styptics of cobweb, hare's fur, dust, etc., that were so popular before the time of Paracelsus.

Heister (1724) said in discussing the control of hemorrhage after amputation, that the older surgeons and still a few in his day, used the actual cautery applied to the openings of

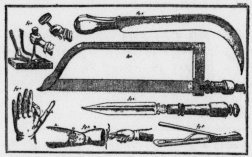

FIG. 14. "BEC DE CORBIN" NOW HOLDS ITSELF CLOSED WITH SPRING (FIG. 6). METHOD OF APPLICATION AND TOURNIQUET ARE SHOWN. (HEISTER, 1718.)

the blood vessels but that this had been largely discarded, partly because of the fear of the patient having a secondary hemorrhage when the eschar over the vessel fell off. He considered the method still useful and safe for the smaller vessels, but many even here he ligated and with greater safety by drawing the vessel out with a "raven's beak" or artery forceps and tying with a strong waxed thread.

In Mr. Cheselden's edition of Le Dran's "The Operations in Surgery" the control of hemorrhage in amputation is discussed as follows:

The hemorrhage may be stopt by different methods, as First, by the application of a button of vitriol to the vessel; Secondly, by applying a button of alum; Thirdly, by a ligature; Each of which has its advantages and inconveniences. The button of vitriol supported by compression is a good way; the vitriol dissolving gradually, cauterizes the vessel and the flesh to a certain height, and the blood coagulating in the vessel above the part cauterized, the eschar falls off by suppuration. This method, however, is not without inconveniences; for if the button of vitriol be too large, the eschar extends farther than we would have it, cauterizing a great deal of the flesh, and sometimes the surface of the bone. To prevent this accident, the button should be very small and well supported. The button of alum, supported likewise by compression, serves equally well to restrain the haemorrhage, by closing the mouth of the vessel, where a clot is formed, which stops the aperture

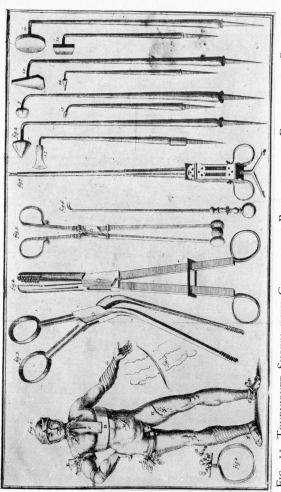

Fig. 15. Tourniquet Shown with Compression Bolsters over Femoral and Brachial Arteries. Cauteries Still Present However. (Heister.)

in the artery; but as it produces no eschar, there is always room to fear that the clot, having nothing to keep it up, may come away, and consequently a haemorrhage ensue. Tying the vessel then is the most secure way; though that too is attended with an inconvenience, it being very difficult to avoid tying the nerve that accompanies the artery, which after a few days sometimes brings on convulsions that make it necessary to cut the ligature.

However, though each of these methods have their inconvenience, yet we are obliged to make use of one of them; and herein we must be determined according as different circumstances appear to make either of them preferable. When a patient is properly accommodated, and can be kept quiet, the button may be applied, as we may thereby secure the haemorrhage without running the hazard of convulsions; but if the patient must be moved after the amputation, it will be proper to use the ligature as being the most secure means, and especially as the convulsions, if they do ensue, do not appear till some days after the operation.

In order to make the ligature, I take a crooked blunt-pointed needle armed with two or three threads waxed together, and pass it round the vessel, taking flesh enough with it to prevent the threads from cutting through. I then tye the two ends of the threads together with a double knot, and make a single once over that. If several vessels bleed together, they must be tied one after another unless they can all be included within the same ligature. This done, the tourniquet is to be loosened entirely, and the ends of the threads should be left long enough to be brought over the stump, that they may be distinguished from the lint which is to cover the wound.

This represents the best practice in the first half of the eighteenth century.

Sharp, a pupil of Cheselden's, in a "Critical Enquiry into the Present State of Surgery" (1750) criticized the current objections to the use of the ligature. He dwelt upon the danger of secondary hemorrhage from the cauterized vessel, believed this even greater in the case of the potential cautery, but in particular he devoted considerable space to the argument that the tying of a nerve would lead to convulsions, a matter stated as a fact by most writers of the time. This was an old doctrine, foisted upon the world by Galen, and persisting today in the vulgar conception that tetanus is the result of an injury to a nerve. He said that though surgeons laid most emphasis on the danger of tying the nerve, large vessels with the accompanying nerve had been ligated many times without producing convulsions and cited Valsalva as having described the dissection of such a double ligation at the elbow. Mass ligation of vessels was now given up partly because of the likelihood of including the adjacent nerves and partly because an attempt was now being made to obtain healing of the wound by something approximating first intention. For the latter purpose, it was advisable to have the ligature come away more quickly, which it did when applied to the vessel alone.

With the crude forceps of the day, designed for the extraction of foreign bodies and resembling the sequestrum forceps of the present time, it was difficult to draw out the artery alone. To meet this need the tenaculum of the ancient Romans was reintroduced and toward the middle of the eighteenth century the policy of careful ligation of all vessels, thus caught up and carefully isolated, was in general use by such men as Desault, Cheselden and Pott.

Down to the end of this century the majority of men thought of the great vessels as powerful agents of possible disaster which needed strong ligatures for their subjugation and the material, whether silk or flax, was gross. Thus a large amount of material was left in the wound. Since the time of Harvey it had gradually become understood that the flow of the blood was outward through the artery and inward through the vein. From both clinical and experimental evidence, it was supposed that pressure in the artery was high and in the vein, low. An exact knowledge of the pressure in these vessels was provided by Stephen Hales in his "Hemadynamics" (1733), in which he described placing a long glass tube in the carotid of a horse and determining the length to which the column of blood rose. Up to this time, also, it was supposed that the arrest of hemorrhage in a divided vessel was in large part mechanical. Coagulation was recognized but thought of more as a result than as the cause of the stoppage of the flow. Petit, who is better known for his tourniquet, studied this topic in 1731 and concluded that the bleeding from a divided artery was stopped by the formation of a coagulum of blood which was situated partly within and partly without the vessel and which adhered to the inside of the artery, to the orifice and to the surrounding parts. After ligation a similar clot formed above the ligature and the same result might be caused by the temporary compression of a vessel. He, for the first time, recognized that the essential factor in the control of hemorrhage was the coagulation of the blood. His conclusions were sharply questioned by those who believed that the constriction and retraction of the artery in a purely mechanical fashion closed the vessel and by others who thought that the swelling of the injured tissue was the important factor. This question was not decided conclusively until the experimental work of Jones, who, trained in the Hunterian school of experimentation, wrote a conclusive monograph on the subject. He was aided in part no doubt by the classical work of William Hewson published as an "Experimental Inquiry into the Properties of the Blood" (1771) in which was described the separation of a "coagulable lymph" from the blood itself. The more detailed anatomical research of the day made possible in part by the more general use of the microscope (Malpighi and van Leeuwenhoek) had demonstrated the three layers of the artery. Desault had previously described the rupture of the inner and middle coats of the artery on ligation. Jones by his experimental work confirmed this. He also clearly demonstrated that the coagulum formed as a result of the rupture of these coats was the essential factor in the staying of hemorrhage. One has but to read the discussion of these points in Cooper's dictionary to realize how the atmosphere was cleared by this experimental work.

Precisely what happened to the ligature was also determined. "Ulceration" in the language of the day occurred through the outer coat, which alone was held within its grasp, the inner and middle having fused with the coagulum and when this ulceration had sufficiently progressed, the thread was released and came away. This process, we now know, was usually the result of sepsis, which did not as a rule invade the inner coats because of the barrier of the intact outer layer. It sometimes did, however, and then separation of the ligature was followed by a secondary hemorrhage, the "bête noir" of the period. It was noted that the greater the amount of suppuration the greater the chance of this happening and in general also, that the degree of suppuration was in direct proportion to the amount of foreign matter left in the wound. In order to lessen this the practice of removing both ends of the ligatures close to the knot was published by Hare in England in 1786. This was never seriously adopted, for the buried knots were invariably discharged from the wound a long time after the healing had been apparently completed. However, the practice revived by Vetch in 1806 of removing one of the threads while leaving the other hanging out of the wound was fairly generally used. In this way the danger of secondary hemorrhage was reduced to a minimum.

It must not be supposed that suppuration of the amputated stump or of the wound was the inevitable result of every operation. The English

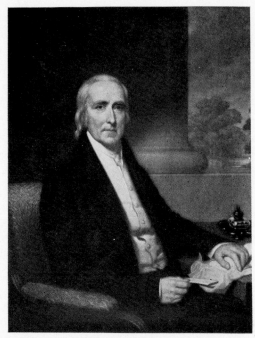

Fig. 16. Philip Syng Physick.

school in particular, following the
lead of Cheselden, strove to obtain
per primam healing. Cleanliness in
every detail was emphasized and the
immediate closure of the wound
attempted, so that frequently, perhaps
as a rule in certain hands, the wound
healed with the exception of the tracts
through which ran the trailing ligatures. If these could be done away
with, then the whole wound might
heal in the desired manner. It is to
the credit of American surgery that
this was seriously attempted and along
the line which later proved successful.
Philip Syng Physick in 1806 recommended and used buckskin twisted in
the form of a thread and with the
ends cut short. The procedure was
described in Dorsey's American
edition of Cooper's surgery and
undoubtedly achieved a considerable
popularity in this country, inasmuch
as Jameson of Baltimore was still
advocating a modification of it in
1827. Nathan Smith employed a buckskin thong in tying the pedicle in his

ovariotomy in 1821 and Ephraim McDowell is said to have employed a similar technique. In England Sir Astley Cooper tried out the procedure but it had apparently fallen into disuse by the time of Liston in 1838, although Malgaigne in France still advocated it. Liston in his "Practical Surgery" says:

The practice of cutting off both ends of the ligature was at one time very much in fashion. It was thought that the mere noose or knot might by possibility remain imbedded in the living tissues, surrounded by a cellular cyst, and occasion no annoyance; and again it was fondly imagined and hoped, that by employing ligatures of animal substance, tendon, cat-gut, or fish-skin, that the noose after answering its purpose of closing the vessel for a sufficient length of time, might be removed by the absorbents, and thus occasion neither irritation nor annoyance. It has never yet been explained, however, by the advocates for this practice, why the absorption of the ligature should take place exactly at the favourable period and not before. Nor has it been shown that it does so at any period, whatever the substance employed may have been. All these hopes have been disappointed; ligatures, of whatever substance, do now and then remain hid for a long time, but very generally they occasion trouble; they, perhaps, after the cure has been thought complete, give rise to irritation, pain, inflammatory swelling and formation of matter; abscess after abscess ensues, one knot comes out after another, and ultimately all the offending foreign bodies may be expelled, but the perfect recovery is thus very long protracted.

IX

THE HEMOSTAT

In the first half of the nineteenth
century with the advance of knowledge concerning the anatomy and
physiology of the blood vessels and its
application, surgeons ventured upon
elective operations, gradually extend-
ing these to a point where the penalty
of sepsis became too great a hazard.
The experimental demonstration by
John Hunter of the development of a
collateral circulation following the
ligation of a vessel led to the elective
ligation in continuity. The immediate
application was to aneurysms of the
peripheral vessels. With the skill
acquired from this experience surgeons became more daring as told in
Halsted's "Operative Story of
Goitre." For instance, occasional mas-
ters attempted extirpation of the
thyroid, the most vascular of all

operative procedures. Von Graefe in Berlin, 1822, removed a thyroid with the ligation of 53 arteries, Roux in 1835 with 47 ligations; Pirogoff in 1849 with a ligation of 30 arteries. General opinion was against this operation, however, and it remained for von Bruns, Kocher and Halsted to perfect the details of the procedure sufficiently to make it reasonably safe. A more profound and accurate knowledge of the blood supply of the gland was needed and some more facile instrument for temporarily arresting hemorrhage than the tenaculum or the ligature carrier.

The invention of the progenitor of the artery forceps, the dental forceps, probably antedates written history. Krombholz says that Erasistratus described a leaden forceps hanging in the temple of the oracle at Delphi. Hippocrates speaks of such an instrument as a necessity for the extraction of teeth and they have been found many times in the armamentarium of the Roman surgeon.

Such instruments were undoubtedly early adopted for the extraction of foreign bodies such as arrowheads and later, missiles thrown by exploding gunpowder. In Albucasis several varieties were depicted and were copied freely down to the time of Paré and Scultetus. The former gives the first description of the application of the forceps to blood vessels when he recommends the use of a "bec de corbin" for drawing out the artery to be ligated. This instrument, modeled on one depicted in Albucasis, was very similar to those found at Pompeii and was used ordinarily for the extraction of foreign bodies as is illustrated elsewhere in Paré's work. In the "Armamentarium Chirurgicum" (1653) of Scultetus, this instrument as well as several others of a similar nature are shown. Down to the time of Desault the vessel was caught necessarily together with surrounding tissue with similar crude and cumbersome instruments or directly in the fingers of the operator or an assistant.

With the development of the practice of carefully isolating the vessels as initiated by Desault in France, and in England by Cheselden, it became important to employ some finer instrument and the tenaculum was resorted to. The antecedents of this likewise fade into the past. We only know that Celsus recommended it for lifting vessels in a wound, so that they might be ligated and Heliodorus for catching them up in the operation for hernia in order to submit them to torsion. It, like the foreign body forceps, has been repeatedly found in the Roman surgical chest. In its rejuvenation as a well fashioned, graceful instrument of precision, it was to appear, next to the knife, as the chief instrument on the surgeon's table until nearly the end of the nineteenth century and in the dexterous hands of such a man as Liston it undoubtedly was most efficient. It was soon modified to become a ligature carrier, the "tertium necessitatum" for the control of hemorrhage during this period.

With the extension of fine dissecting in human and comparative anatomy and the manipulation of microscopical objects, there developed the dissecting forceps, such as is still used. This with a contrivance for holding it closed as suggested by von Graefe, the elder, became the first instrument properly called the artery forceps. Amussat of Paris, at about the same time (1829) devised a similar device for torsion of the vessels while Bushe of New York checked bleeding "by twisting the cut extremities of the vessels in a square beaked forceps, furnished with a sliding bar and two nuts."

Mr. Liston in 1838 said:

If the cellular substance is loose and fine, no difficulty will be experienced in pulling out the open end of the vessel, by the use of the common dissection forceps, or sharp hook tenaculum as it is commonly called. When no assistance is at hand, the surgeon will find the advantage

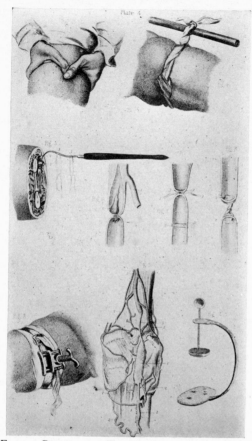

FIG. 17. PRACTICE OF TOURNIQUET AND TENACULUM
AS DEPICTED IN SMITH (1850).

of possessing a pair of forceps with well fitted joints and which are held closely in contact by a catch or slide; these are now to be had of the various instrument makers, of a much less clumsy form than heretofore.

For amputation through the thigh his instrumentarium consisted of: "a long, narrow, blunt-backed and sharp-pointed knife, a plain, good, and serviceable saw, a pair of dissecting forceps and *a pair or two with a catch.*" No tenaculum was included, apparently because he had come to rely upon the forceps which were to bear his name in English literature down to the present time. In Smith's "System of Surgery" (1850), an excellent steel engraving shows such forceps and also the progenitor of our modern hemostat, Philip Syng Physick's artery clamp and needle holder invented in 1800, while below it is shown the bullet forceps from which it was very apparently an offspring of the first generation. It only needed the addition of a ratchet instead of a hook-catch to make it quite modern.

Probably with knowledge of this, Charriere in 1858 introduced a similar forceps with a catch and ring handle for dressings and for the torsion of vessels. In 1862, Koeberlé used these for clamping a vessel, leaving them in place for several days, the principle being somewhat similar to Sir James Simpson's acupressure of the same period. Péan in 1867 and Spencer Wells in 1872 popularized this forci-pressure and each devised hemostatic clamps which still survive under their respective names. At the same time, these clamps and a similar one, described by Bryant, were used largely for the torsion of vessels without tying and with surprising success, even arteries the size of the femoral being so controlled.

Halsted gives a description of von Bruns' methods as reported by Suskind in 1877:

The tissues to be divided were canalized layerwise with Cooper's scissors, the

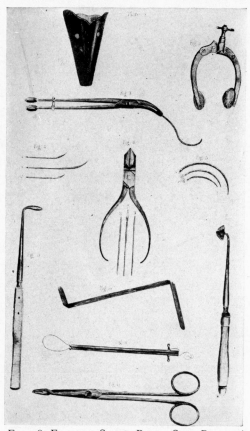

FIG. 18. FIGURE 3 SHOWS PHILIP SYNG PHYSICK'S
NEEDLE HOLDER AND FIGURE 12 A FORCEPS, WHICH
WITH CATCH WOULD BE PRACTICALLY MODERN.
CAUTERY HAS ALMOST GONE. (SMITH, 1850.)

fingers or the handle of a knife. Along the passage thus made, a ligature-needle would be passed, and the tissues, including vessels, would be divided between the two ligatures.

I was pleased to find in Suskind's description a list of instruments employed by Bruns in his operations for goitre: "Several pointed bistouries, several forceps (preferably toothed forceps), Cooper's scissors, one aneurism-needle (preferably the blunt, ligation-needle of Bruns), a Muzeux's hooked forceps (Vulsella) or a fenestrated forceps, ligature-rods of Graefe or Dupuytren, catgut and silk, sponges, water, blunt hooks." No mention is made of artery forceps; this may be an oversight, for Bruns in his Handbuch der Chirurgischen Praxis, vol. i, p. 29 (1873) says: "The ordinary forceps which are closed by finger pressure can be held permanently closed by various devices, among which the Schiebervorrichtung of Fricke has proved to be best suited to the purpose. Most frequently such lockable forceps are employed for the tying of bleeding arteries and hence have been named artery forceps, although they are often used to grasp the cut edges of the skin or mucous membrane, or bits of sponge with which blood and mucous are wiped away."

Halsted remarks of Billroth's clinic at the same period:

Clamps had come into use and Billroth was evidently learning some of the various purposes which they were to serve; for example, he divided tissues containing vessels between two of them and would leave a number hanging in the wound.

The development of the modern hemostat is best given in Halsted's own words:

On my return from Germany in 1881, I was impressed with the fact that our surgeons were greatly handicapped in most of their operations by lack of proper instruments, particularly of artery clamps. These were insufficient in number and faulty in design. In most of the New York Hospitals the only artery clamps were of the fenestrated, mouse-toothed, spring forceps variety (Liston's and Wakley's), indeed, these were about the only ones procurable either in this country or

England. In the elaborate catalogue for
1882 of S. Maw, Son and Thompson, London, no other artery forceps, torsion forceps excepted, is mentioned.

In a catalogue of Collins et Cie, Paris,
undated, but evidently of about the same
period, the little artery clamps of Koeberle and of Pean are the only ones
figured; "pinces à arteres à ressorts" are
catalogued, the latter probably being the
mouse-toothed forceps given in the London catalogue (Maw and Son) and quite
universally employed in America until
1880 or a little later. In Gunther's
Surgery (vol. i, Plate 5, opp. p. 36) is a
remarkable lithograph which indicates the
part played by the tenaculum in
hemostasis in 1859. The divided artery,
open-mouthed, is hooked up on the point
of the instrument, the handle of which is
held in the mouth of the operator who,
evidently, was shorthanded. Until about
1890, the tenaculum was a favorite instrument in America for checking hemorrhage,
especially with some of the senior surgeons,
and until about 1880 was quite universally employed here, its only rivals being
the inadequate mouse-toothed, spring
forceps and the Pean or Koeberle clamps.

Then almost simultaneously came the clamps of Spencer Wells and (1879) of the writer, of which the Pean-Koeberle clamp was the prototype. The point of my clamp was snub-nosed originally, but the length and spread of the handles, the essentially new features, were the same as at present. With the development of the transfixion method with milliner's needles and use of the fine black silk, the nose of the clamp was made finer (1889). Two or three years later it assumed its present form. Rarely had I seen in our country, prior to my first visit to Europe (1879), more than one artery clamp at a time left hanging in a wound. Clamps were too few for this —four to three or even two being considered ample for an operation. Few hospitals, in New York at least, possessed as many as six artery clamps in 1880. I recall vividly an operation in Vienna performed by Mikulicz in 1879 in Billroth's clinic. Americans, newly arrived in Austria, we were greatly amused at seeing perhaps a dozen clamps (Schieber) left hanging in a wound of the neck while the operator proceeded with his dissection, and were inclined to ridicule the method as being untidy or uncouth. Slowly it dawned upon us that we in America were novices in the art as well as the science of surgery. The artery forceps, adequate in number and design, undoubtedly played a very important rôle in the strikingly rapid progress in the art of operating made by surgeons, the world over, in the final quarter of the past century. The value of the artery clamps is not likely to be overestimated. They determine methods and effect results impossible without them. They tranquilize the operator. In a wound that is perfectly dry, and in tissues never permitted to become even stained by blood, the operator, unperturbed, may work for hours without fatigue. The confidence gradually acquired from masterfulness in controlling hemorrhage gives to the surgeon the calm which is so essential for clear thinking and orderly procedure at the operating table.

X

LISTER AND THE LIGATURE

The development of the artery forceps was occasioned by the great increase in the volume of surgery which was the result of the introduction of anesthesia in 1846 and of the Listerian principles of 1865 to 1870. The latter also had a profound influence on the mode of use and the material of the ligature in which Lister's contribution was only second to that of the introduction of his antiseptic method.

With previous attempts to obtain early and complete healing of the wound by the cutting off of the ends of the ligatures, the knots came away in repeated sinuses and delayed the time of healing. This was true even with the animal ligatures proposed by Physick, yet they had not completely

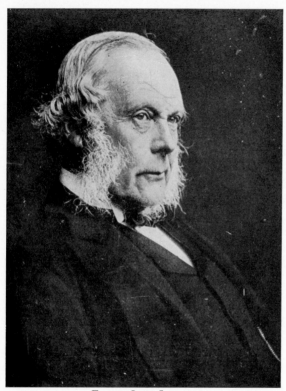

FIG. 19. LORD LISTER.

gone out of practice for Malgaigne in 1852 still said:

We prefer the ligature of doe-skin, not soft, as Jameson likes them, but rolled up, as used by Physick and Dorsey. They divide the inner coat like vegetable thread but are easily absorbed, so that we may remove the two extremities very near the knot; if on the contrary common thread is used, only one end is cut, and the other hangs from the wound.

In 1867 Lister in his second paper on "The Antiseptic Principle" indicated that he was already experimenting with the ligature:

On the 12th of December last, I tied the left carotid of a horse about the middle of the neck, using fine but strong "purse-silk," unwaxed, but steeped for some time in a saturated watery solution of carbolic acid. The ligature having been tightly tied, so as to rupture the internal and middle coats, its ends were cut short, and the wound was freely treated with carbolic acid dissolved in forty parts of water.

Demonstrating the specimen later removed, he noted that the thread had been bridged over externally by dense fibrous tissues. He felt that this demonstrated: "that the antiseptic system would free the deligation of a large artery in its continuity of the two essential elements of danger to which it is now liable, viz., an unhealthy condition of the wound and secondary haemorrhage."

He at once carried the conclusions arrived at from this experiment into practice and in January of that year ligated the external iliac for an aneurysm of the femoral artery, using twisted silk which had been soaked in carbolic acid, the operation being conducted throughout according to the antiseptic method. Unfortunately, he had not yet learned that the wound should be closed completely and he introduced a "pledget of lint" deeply into it, projecting externally to act as a drain. At the end of a fortnight the last of the lint was removed and in four weeks the wound was completely cicatrized. Ten months later the patient died from the rupture of a thoracic aneurysm and Lister was enabled to examine the results of the operation. He found that:

At the narrowest part the artery was reduced to mere fibrous tissue, constituting a dense white band five-eighths of an inch long, from the middle of which was seen projecting at one side a round, buff-coloured appendage about a line in diameter, somewhat obscured by a trifling amount of inflammatory condensation of texture in the immediate vicinity. On scratching this little body with the point of a knife, I found it to be a very thin-walled capsule, containing the knot of the ligature, with two tapering ends, which were shorter than the thread was cut at the operation, while the noose had vanished altogether. The surface of the knot also showed clear indications of having been subjected to an eroding agency, similar, no doubt, to that exerted by granulations upon dead bone absorbed by them. Besides the remnant of the ligature, the tiny capsule contained a minute quantity of yellowish, semifluid material, looking to the naked eye like very thick pus. There can be no doubt that the presence of the thread was in some way or other the cause of this and I think we can hardly be wrong in assuming that, in order to give rise to such degeneration of tissue, it must have operated as a persistent, if trifling, source of abnormal stimulation. Now, as putrefaction is here out of the question, and as the substance of silk is not chemically stimulating, we seem shut up to the conclusion that the thread must have occasioned disturbance of a mechanical nature.

Not having at hand cultural methods to be developed shortly by Pasteur and Koch, no attempt was made to grow organisms from this pus and Lister assumed that silk as a material must be discarded because it produced mechanical irritation. We now know that his conclusions were wrong and that he was dealing with an infected ligature probably via the lint drain. This led him to turn to the "animal" or absorbable ligature as a solution of the problem. He discussed this as follows:

The use of "animal ligatures," of catgut, leather, or tendon, was long since
tried and abandoned as unsatisfactory;
but after the experience which the antiseptic system has afforded of the disap-
pearance, without suppuration, of large
dead pieces of skin and other textures,
there could be little doubt that threads of
animal tissue, if applied antiseptically,
would be similarly disposed of.

On the 31st of December, 1868, I tied
the right carotid artery about the middle
of the neck in a healthy calf a few days
old, the animal being under chloroform.
Ligatures of two different kinds were
employed, at an interval of about an inch
and a half, the sheath of the vessel being
left undisturbed in the intervening part.
The cardiac ligature was of home manufacture, composed of three strips of
peritoneum from the small intestine of an
ox, firmly twisted together into a three-
fold cord. The distal thread was of fine
catgut, called "minikin gut" by the London makers. Both had been soaked for
four hours in a saturated watery solution
of carbolic acid, which swelled and softened them, so that the thread of my own
making was too large to enter the eye of

the aneurysm-needle except near the ends, where it was thinner than elsewhere. This substantial ligature, bore the strain of tying well, but the fine catgut broke as I tightened the noose. I did not, however, remove it, but having a second piece at my disposal, passed it round at the same place, and with gentle traction completed the knot. There were thus two ligatures of the fine gut at the distal site. All were cut short except one end of the catgut, which I purposely left about three-quarters of an inch long, to give a better opportunity of ascertaining what would become of the foreign method.

He then described how living tissue grew into the crust in a wound and continued:

Hence it might have been anticipated that the ligatures of peritoneum and catgut placed on the calf's carotid would, after the expiration of a month, be found transformed into bands of living tissue. Such was, in truth, the case, as was apparent on closer examination. They had, indeed, a deceptive resemblance to their former condition, from the persistence in their substance of the impurities

of the original materials, the dark adventi-
tious particles being of mineral nature
incapable of absorption, so that they had
remained as a sort of tatooing of the new
structure. Nevertheless, a marked altera-
tion in colour had taken place, especially
in the distal ligature, where the dirty grey
of the softened catgut had changed to a
dirty pink tint. The two pieces of catgut
which had been tied around the vessel at
that part had become, as it were, fused
together into a single fleshy band, insepa-
rably blended with the external coat of the
artery. The knots were nowhere discover-
able, and the only indication of the end
which had been left long at the time of the
operation was the presence of a black
speck here and there upon a delicate
thread of cellular tissue in connexion
with the vessel.

He described the microscopical
reaction and called attention to the
fibroplastic reaction of tissues which
invaded the ligature. In conclusion, he
said:

It appears, then, that by applying a
ligature of animal tissue antiseptically
upon an artery, whether tightly or gently,

we virtually surround it with a ring of living tissue, and strengthen the vessel where we obstruct it. The surgeon, therefore, may now tie an arterial trunk in its continuity close to a large branch, secure alike against secondary haemorrhage and deep-seated suppuration—provided always that he has so studied the principles of the antiseptic system, and so carefully considered the details of the mode of dressing best adapted to the particular case in hand, that he can feel certain of avoiding putrefaction in the wound. For my own part, I should now, without hesitation, undertake ligature of the innominate, believing that it would prove a very safe procedure.

He spoke of the availability of catgut:

. . . catgut, manufactured from the small intestine of the sheep, may be had at a low price, from the thickness of a horsehair upwards. As sold in the shops, however, it is quite unfit for the purpose of the surgeon. For, when moistened with water or with the animal fluids, it becomes not only very soft and weak, but as slippery as a piece of recent intestine, so that a knot tied upon it yields to the slightest traction.

He at once entered upon experimentation as to the manufacture of catgut, first producing a carbolized gut and in 1876 describing its chromatization, the last essential step in the production of the present-day absorbable ligature.

The choice of catgut was in a sense fortuitous. It was and still remains the only absorbable animal tissue in the form of a thread which is a matter of common commerce. Its origin, like that of silk, linen and woolen thread, is lost in antiquity. It was used for the bowstring of the North American Indian and for the primitive stringed musical instruments of the native inhabitants of India. Odysseus stretched the twisted intestine of the sheep upon the bow which gave forth grim music for the suitors of Penelope and the strings of the Egyptian and Greek lyre were of catgut. Indeed, Wilkinson found an instrument so strung in the tomb of Rameses and was able to elicit after some 3000 years a note from the same cord which may have charmed the ear of the great Pharaoh himself. Catgut was to be obtained in Rome, for Galen suggested its use as a substitute for linen and Rhazes used it in the suture of the intestine, perhaps on the principle of *similia similibus curantur*. With the development of the bowed string instrument, the progenitor of the violin, catgut became an important article of commerce in Italy and France. Its sporadic use as a ligature up until the time of Lister must have led, in many instances, to infection of the most disastrous kind, such as anthrax and tetanus, but the discovery of antisepsis and asepsis rendered its use safe. It was rapidly adopted throughout the world.

The art of hemostasis, equalling in importance the control of infection and the introduction of anesthesia, has been slowly but finally learned.

The manipulation of the present day —the application of an artery forceps and the casting about the vessel of a ligature—is so simple a process that we little realize the travail that has gone into its perfection. The groping Alexandrian anatomist, the practical Greco-Roman surgeon, the consummate Paré, the obscure Morel, and the patient experimentalist, Lister, contributed the essentials, a host of surgeons provided the refinements. As a result, the operator of today may relegate to the background of the procedure that which for ages was an almost insurmountable obstacle and proceed without fear of hemorrhage calmly and unhurriedly, in such a manner as to ensure for the patient all that surgical skill can provide.

INDEX OF PERSONAL NAMES

INDEX OF PERSONAL NAMES

INDEX OF PERSONAL NAMES

INDEX OF PERSONAL NAMES

INDEX OF PERSONAL NAMES

SUBJECT INDEX

SUBJECT INDEX

SUBJECT INDEX

SUBJECT INDEX

SUBJECT INDEX